Judith Green

Keto
Cookbook

Quick and Easy Low-Carb
Homemade Recipes

Table of Contents

Introduction

Trying to lose weight, maintain low blood pressure, cure diabetes, and maintain overall body wellness can be quite challenging, especially if you have tried different means without getting the desired result. There are tons of procedures, diets, and ways to lose weight, but only a few of them work. If you ask me, I would tell you how many different methods I've tried to lose weight and maintain overall wellness, and how many of them failed to deliver results but instead led to more complications due to their adverse side effects. However, the Keto diet was a ball game for me. Over time, I was able to lose weight and achieve overall well-being without complications.

If you are trying to lose weight and achieve a healthy overall being without experiencing complications, I would recommend you try the keto diet. It is about the safest, natural, and most effective way to lose weight and achieve the best results in your journey to overall wellness.

What Is Keto Diet?

A keto diet is an eating plan focused on foods that offer a high amount of healthful fat, moderate level of protein, and very low carbohydrates. People who say they are on a 'keto diet' are people who ensure that their regular food intake contains a lot of healthful fat, an adequate amount of protein, and very low carbohydrates. This means their dietary macronutrients are divided into about 55% to 60% fat, 30% to 35% protein, and 5% to 10% carbohydrate. In the end, the goal of the keto diet is to get more energy from healthful fats than from carbohydrates.

How Does It Work?

Your body makes use of any energy source it finds readily available, which is often glucose converted from carbohydrates. By increasing the level of healthful fat you take and reducing your carbohydrate intake, your glycogen level depletes, which forces your body to go through metabolic changes. Two metabolic processes occur when your body stores low-level carbohydrates. They are called gluconeogenesis and ketogenesis. Glycogenesis is the production of glucose in your body, and when the glucose production level stops due to low carbohydrate levels, the production of glucose becomes too low to keep up with the needs of your body, which forces your body to adapt to ketogenesis as an alternative. Ketogenesis begins to produce the energy for your body, and ketone bodies become your body's primary source of energy, which is known as the 'ketosis state' that continues to be as long as your body is deprived of carbohydrates. Because your body is deprived of carbohydrates, which is primarily the cause of weight gain, your body can burn fat faster and convert the available fat into energy.

The ketone bodies are integrated into your body system and are used to produce energy through the heart, muscle tissue, and kidneys and also cross the blood-brain barrier to be an alternative source of energy to the brain.

History and Origin of Keto Diet

The Keto diet was first used to treat epilepsy in 1921 by Russel Wilder, after which it became a widely acceptable dietary therapy to treat epilepsy. However, its popularity ceased after the 1930s due to the introduction of antiepileptic drugs.

The keto diet recently became a widely accepted procedure for weight loss, treatment for diabetes, cancer, and other illnesses and has proven, based on experience and scientific studies, to be safe and highly effective.

How Does Keto Diet Compare to other Diet?

The Keto diet has proven to be a much more effective procedure to achieve weight loss, cure diabetes, control blood sugar levels and maintain an overall healthy body system than a low-fat diet. Here is what research says:

Weight Loss

A review of 13 studies showed that a consistent intake of very low carbohydrates was more effective than undergoing a low-fat diet. Participants who followed the keto diet lost an average of 2 pounds (0.9kg) more than the participants that followed a low-fat diet.
A study carried on 34 older adults found out that the participants who underwent the keto diet for eight weeks lost about five times as much total body fat as those who followed a low-fat diet.

Diabetes

Research conducted by NCBI in 349 participants with type 2 diabetes discovered that those who practiced the keto diet lost an average of 26.2 pounds (11.9kg) in 2 years. The research also noted that those participants also experienced a significant decrease in their blood sugar levels.

Another study conducted by PubMed in 2019 on women with type 2 diabetes discovered that women who practiced the keto diet for 90 days greatly reduced the level of hemoglobin AIC which shows a high level of long-term blood sugar management.

There are tons of studies that have proven the keto diet to be a much more effective way for weight loss, diabetes treatment, control of blood sugar level, and general well-being. But I've only selected a few of them in order not to bore you with too many statistics. If you want to find out more, I encourage you to do further research to make a personal conclusion.

That being said, let's dive into the numerous reasons to adopt the keto diet in the next chapter.

Chapter 1. Breakfast Recipes

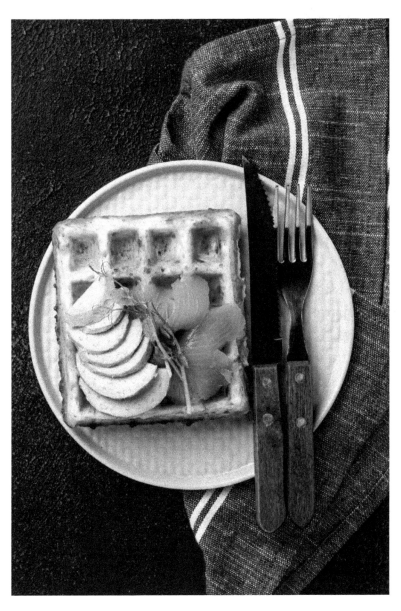

1 Belgium Waffles with Cheese Spread

Total Time: approx. 25 minutes | 2 servings

INGREDIENTS:

½ cup cream cheese, softened

1 lemon, zested and juiced

2 tbsp stevia

2 tbsp olive oil

½ cup almond milk

3 eggs

½ cup almond flour

DIRECTIONS:

In a bowl, combine the cream cheese, lemon juice and zest and stevia.

In a separate bowl, whisk the olive oil, almond milk, and eggs.

Stir in the almond flour and combine until no lumps exist.

Let the batter sit for 5 minutes to thicken.

Spritz a waffle iron with a non-stick cooking spray.

Ladle a ¼ cup of the batter into the waffle iron and cook for about 5 minutes.

Repeat with the remaining batter.

Slice the waffles into quarters; apply the lemon spread in between each of two waffles and snap and serve.

NUTRITION: Cal 322; Fat 26g; Net Carbs 7.7g; Protein 11g

2   Cheese Soufflés

Prep time: 15 minutes | Cook time: 12 minutes |
Serves 4

INGREDIENTS:

3 large eggs, whites and yolks separated

¼ teaspoon cream of tartar

½ cup shredded sharp Cheddar cheese

3 ounces (85 g) cream cheese, softened

DIRECTIONS:

In a large bowl, beat egg whites together with cream of tartar until soft peaks form, about 2 minutes.

In a separate medium bowl, beat egg yolks, Cheddar, and cream cheese together until frothy, about 1 minute. Add egg yolk mixture to whites, gently folding until combined.

Pour mixture evenly into four 4-inch ramekins greased with cooking spray. Place ramekins into air fryer basket. Adjust the temperature to 350°F (180°C) and set the timer for 12 minutes. Eggs will be browned on the top and firm in the center when done. Serve warm.

NUTRITION: Cal: 183 | fat: 14g | protein: 9g | carbs: 1g | net carbs: 1g | fiber: 0g

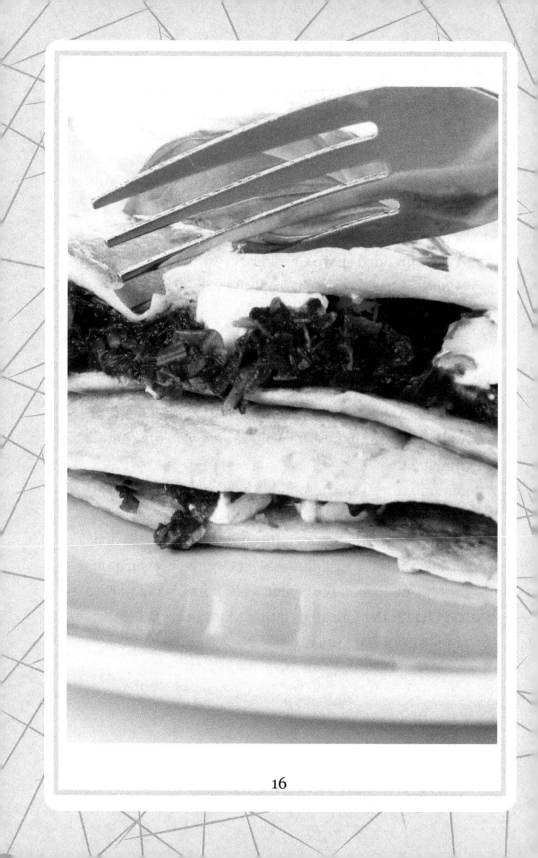

3   Spinach & Feta Cheese Pancakes

Total Time: approx. 10 minutes | 2 servings

INGREDIENTS:

½ cup almond flour

½ tsp baking powder

½ cup feta cheese, crumbled

½ cup spinach, chopped

2 tbsp coconut milk

1 egg

DIRECTIONS:

Beat the egg with a fork in a medium bowl.

Add in the almond flour, baking powder, feta cheese, coconut milk, and spinach; and whisk to combine.

Set a skillet over medium heat and let it heat for a minute.

Fetch a soup spoonful of mixture into the skillet and cook for approximately 2 minutes.

Flip the pancake and cook further for 1 minute.

Remove onto a plate and repeat the cooking process until the batter is exhausted.

Serve with your favorite topping.

NUTRITION: Cal 412; Fat 32g; Net Carbs 5.9g; Protein 12g

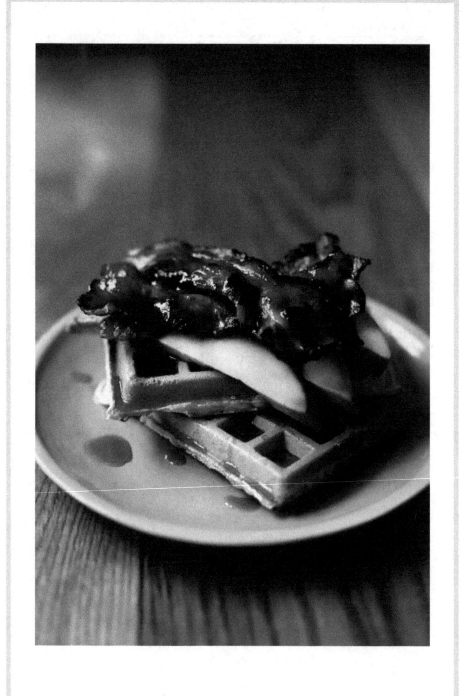

4 Jalapeno Waffles with Bacon & Avocado

Total Time: approx. 20 minutes | 2 servings

INGREDIENTS:

2 tbsp butter, melted

¼ cup almond milk

2 tbsp almond flour

Salt and black pepper to taste

½ tsp parsley, chopped

½ jalapeño pepper, minced

4 eggs

½ cup cheddar, crumbled

4 slices bacon, chopped

1 avocado, sliced

DIRECTIONS:

In a skillet over medium heat, fry bacon until crispy, about 5 minutes.

Remove to a plate.

In a mixing bowl, combine the remaining ingredients, except the avocado.

Preheat a waffle iron and grease with cooking spray.

Pour in the batter and close the lid.

Cook for about 5 minutes or until the desired consistency is reached.

Do the same with the rest of the batter.

Decorate with avocado and bacon.

Serve immediately.

NUTRITION: Cal 771; Fat 67g; Net Carbs 6.9g; Protein 27g

5 Bacon & Cheese Pesto Mug Cakes

Ready in about: 8 minutes | Serves: 2

INGREDIENTS:

Muffin:

¼ cup flax meal

1 egg

2 tbsp heavy cream

2 tbsp pesto

¼ cup almond flour

Salt and black pepper to taste

Filling:

2 tbsp cream cheese

4 slices bacon

½ medium avocado, sliced

DIRECTIONS:

Mix together the dry muffin ingredients in a bowl. Add egg, heavy cream, and pesto, and whisk well with a fork. Season with salt and pepper. Divide the mixture between two ramekins. Place in the microwave and cook for 60-90 seconds. Leave to cool slightly before filling.

Meanwhile, in a skillet, over medium heat, cook the bacon slices until crispy. Transfer to paper towels to soak up excess fat; set aside. Invert the muffins onto a plate and cut in half, crosswise. To assemble the sandwiches: spread cream cheese and top with bacon and avocado slices.

NUTRITION: Cal 511, Fat: 38.2g, Net Carbs: 4.5g, Protein: 16.4g

Chapter 2. Snack & Appetizer Recipes

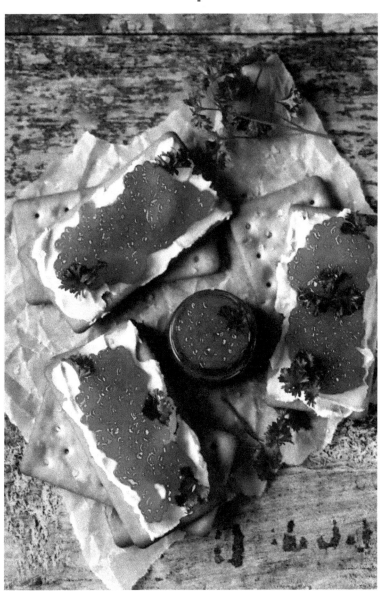

6 Anchovy Fat Bombs

Prep time: 15 minutes | Cook time: 0 minutes | Serves 10

INGREDIENTS:

8 ounces (227 g) Cheddar cheese, shredded

6 ounces (170 g) cream cheese, at room temperature

4 ounces (113 g) canned anchovies, chopped

½ yellow onion, minced

1 teaspoon fresh garlic, minced

Sea salt and ground black pepper, to taste

DIRECTIONS:

Mix all of the above ingredients in a bowl. Place the mixture in your refrigerator for 1 hour.

Then, shape the mixture into bite-sized balls.

Serve immediately.

NUTRITION:

calories: 123 | fat: 8.8g | protein: 7.4g | carbs: 3.3g | net carbs: 3.3g | fiber: 0g

7   Pork and Scallion Meatball

Prep time: 20 minutes | Cook time: 18 minutes | Serves 8

INGREDIENTS:

½ teaspoon fine sea salt

1 cup Romano cheese, grated

3 cloves garlic, minced

1½ pounds (680g) ground pork

½ cup scallions, finely chopped

2 eggs, well whisked

⅓ teaspoon cumin powder

⅔ teaspoon ground black pepper, or more to taste

2 teaspoons basil

DIRECTIONS:

Simply combine all the ingredients in a large-sized mixing bowl.

Shape into bite-sized balls; cook the meatballs in the air fryer for 18 minutes at 345°F (174°C). Serve with some tangy sauce such as marinara sauce if desired. Bon appétit!

NUTRITION:

calories: 350 | fat: 25g | protein: 28g | carbs: 2g | net carbs: 1g | fiber: 1g

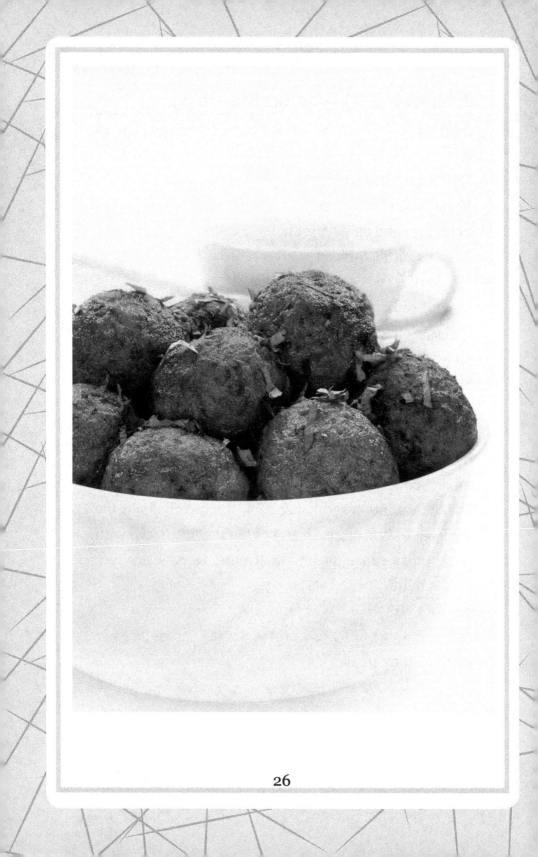

8 Mustard-Cayenne Pork Meatballs

Prep time: 25 minutes | Cook time: 17 minutes |
Serves 8

INGREDIENTS:

1 teaspoon cayenne pepper

2 teaspoons mustard

2 tablespoons Brie cheese, grated

5 garlic cloves, minced

2 small-sized yellow onions, peeled and chopped

1½ pounds (680g) ground pork

Sea salt and freshly ground black pepper, to taste

DIRECTIONS:

Mix all of the above ingredients until everything is well incorporated.

Now, form the mixture into balls (the size of golf a ball).
Cook for 17 minutes at 375°F (190°C). Serve with your favorite sauce.

NUTRITION:

calories: 275 | fat: 18g | protein: 3g | carbs: 3g | net carbs: 2g | fiber: 1g

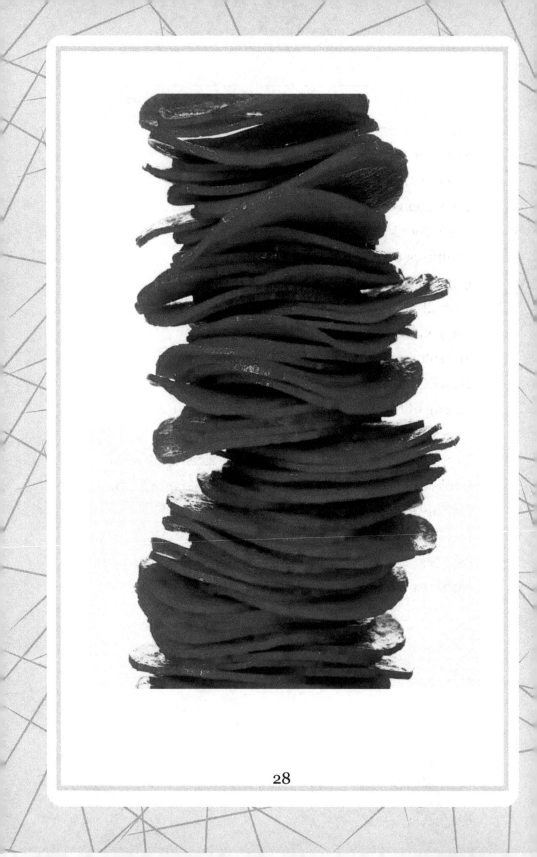

9   Crispy Pepperoni

Prep time: 5 minutes | Cook time: 8 minutes | Serves 2

INGREDIENTS:

14 slices pepperoni

DIRECTIONS:

Place pepperoni slices into ungreased air fryer basket. Adjust the temperature to 350°F (180°C) and set the timer for 8 minutes. Pepperoni will be browned and crispy when done. Let cool 5 minutes before serving. Store in airtight container at room temperature up to 3 days.

NUTRITION:

calories: 69 | fat: 5g | protein: 3g | carbs: 0g | net carbs: 0g | fiber: 0g

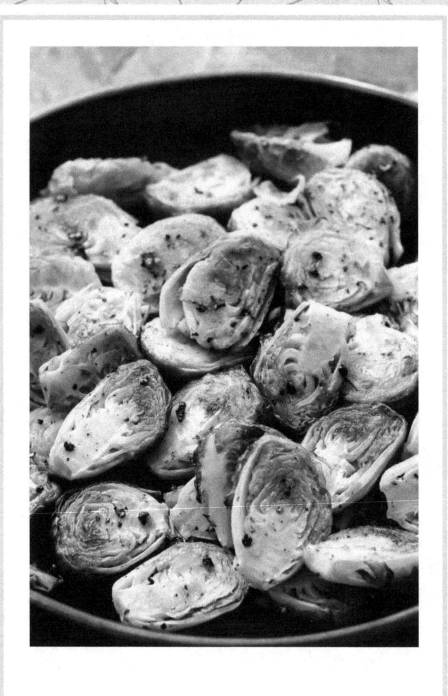

10 Brussels Sprouts with Fennel Seeds

Prep time: 20 minutes | Cook time: 15 minutes |
Serves 4

INGREDIENTS:

1 pound (454 g) Brussels sprouts, ends and yellow
leaves removed and halved lengthwise

Salt and black pepper, to taste

1 tablespoon toasted sesame oil

1 teaspoon fennel seeds

Chopped fresh parsley, for garnish

DIRECTIONS:

Place the Brussels sprouts, salt, pepper, sesame oil, and
fennel seeds in a resealable plastic bag. Seal the bag
and shake to coat.

Air-fry at 380°F (193°C) for 15 minutes or until tender.
Make sure to flip them over halfway through the
cooking time.

Serve sprinkled with fresh parsley. Bon appétit!

NUTRITION:

calories: 174 | fat: 3g | protein: 3g | carbs: 9g | net
carbs: 5g | fiber: 4g

Chapter 3. Poultry Recipes

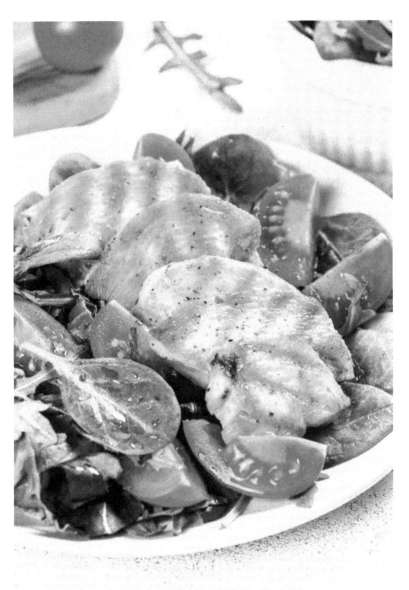

11 Garlic & Ginger Chicken with Peanut Sauce

Ready in about: 20 minutes + marinating time |
Serves: 6

INGREDIENTS:

Chicken ingredients

1 tbsp wheat-free soy sauce

1 tbsp sugar-free fish sauce

1 tbsp lime juice

1 tsp cilantro, chopped

1 minced garlic

1 tsp minced ginger

1 tbsp olive oil

1 tbsp rice wine vinegar

1 tsp cayenne pepper

1 tbsp erythritol

6 chicken thighs

Peanut sauce

½ cup peanut butter

1 tsp minced garlic

1 tbsp lime juice

2 tbsp water

1 tsp minced ginger

1 tbsp jalapeño pepper, chopped

2 tbsp rice wine vinegar

2 tbsp erythritol

1 tbsp fish sauce

DIRECTIONS:

Combine all chicken ingredients in a large Ziploc bag. Seal the bag and shake to combine. Refrigerate for 1 hour. Remove from the fridge about 15 minutes before cooking. Preheat the grill to medium heat.

Cook the chicken for 7 minutes per side until golden brown. Remove to a serving plate. Whisk together all the sauce ingredients in a mixing bowl. Serve the chicken drizzled with peanut sauce.

NUTRITION: Cal 492, Fat: 36g, Net Carbs: 3g, Protein: 35g

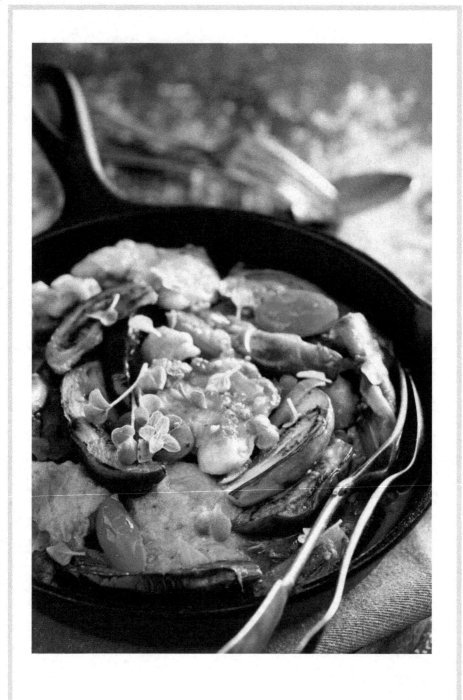

12 Eggplant & Tomato Braised Chicken Thighs

Ready in about: 45 minutes | Serves: 4

INGREDIENTS:

2 tbsp ghee

1 lb chicken thighs

Salt and black pepper to taste

2 garlic cloves, minced

1 (14 oz) can whole tomatoes

1 eggplant, diced

DIRECTIONS:

Melt ghee in a saucepan over medium heat. Season the chicken with salt and black pepper and fry for 4 minutes on each side until golden brown. Remove to a plate. Sauté the garlic in the ghee for 2 minutes.

Pour in the tomatoes and cook covered for 8 minutes. Add in the eggplant and sauté for 4 minutes. Adjust the seasoning with salt and black pepper. Stir and add the chicken. Coat with sauce and simmer for 3 minutes. Serve chicken with sauce on a bed of squash pasta.

NUTRITION: Cal 468, Fat 39.5g, Net Carbs 2g, Protein 26g

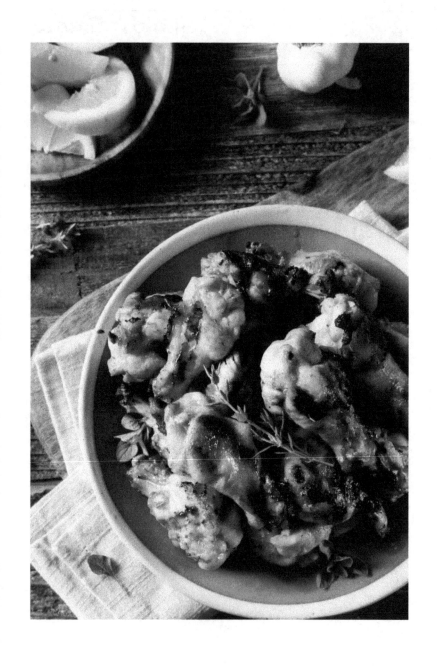

13 Lemon-Garlic Chicken Skewers

Ready in about: 20 minutes + marinating time | Serves: 4

INGREDIENTS:

1 lb chicken breasts, cut into cubes

2 tbsp olive oil

2/3 jar preserved lemon, drained

2 garlic cloves, minced

½ cup lemon juice

Salt and black pepper to taste

1 tsp fresh rosemary, chopped

4 lemon wedges

DIRECTIONS:

In a wide bowl, mix half of the oil, garlic, salt, pepper, and lemon juice and add the chicken cubes and lemon rind. Let marinate for 2 hours in the refrigerator. Remove the chicken and thread it onto skewers.

Heat a grill pan over high heat. Add in the chicken skewers and sear them for 6 minutes per side. Remove to a plate and serve warm garnished with rosemary and lemons wedges.

NUTRITION: Cal 350, Fat 11g, Net Carbs 3.5g, Protein 34g

14 Sweet Chili Grilled Chicken

Ready in about: 30 minutes | Serves: 6

INGREDIENTS:

2 lb chicken breasts

4 cloves garlic, minced

2 tbsp fresh oregano, chopped

½ cup lemon juice

2/3 cup olive oil

1 tbsp erythritol

Salt and black pepper to taste

3 small chilies, minced

DIRECTIONS:

Preheat grill to high heat. In a bowl, mix the garlic, oregano, lemon juice, olive oil, chilies, and erythritol. Cover the chicken with plastic wraps and use the rolling pin to pound to ½-inch thickness.

Remove the wrap and brush the spice mixture on the chicken on all sides. Place on the grill and cook for 15 minutes, flip, and continue cooking for 10 more minutes. Remove to a plate and serve with salad.

NUTRITION: Cal 265, Fat 9g, Net Carbs 3g, Protein 26g

15   Turkey Chorizo with Bok Choy

Ready in about 50 minutes | Servings 4

INGREDIENTS:

4 mild turkey Chorizo, sliced 1/2 cup full-fat milk 6 ounces Gruyère cheese, preferably freshly grated 1 yellow onion, chopped Coarse salt and ground black pepper, to taste 1 pound Bok choy, tough stem ends trimmed 1 cup cream of mushroom soup 1 tablespoon lard, room temperature

DIRECTIONS:

Melt the lard in a nonstick skillet over a moderate flame; cook the Chorizo sausage for about 5 minutes, stirring occasionally to ensure even cooking; reserve. Add in the onion, salt, pepper, Bok choy, and cream of mushroom soup. Continue to cook for 4 minutes longer or until the vegetables have softened. Spoon the mixture into a lightly oiled casserole dish. Top with the reserved Chorizo. In a mixing bowl, thoroughly combine the milk and cheese. Pour the cheese mixture over the sausage. Cover with foil and bake at 365 degrees F for about 35 minutes.Enjoy!

NUTRITION: 189 Calories; 12g Fat; 2.6g Carbs; 9.4g Protein; 1g Fiber

Chapter 4. Beef

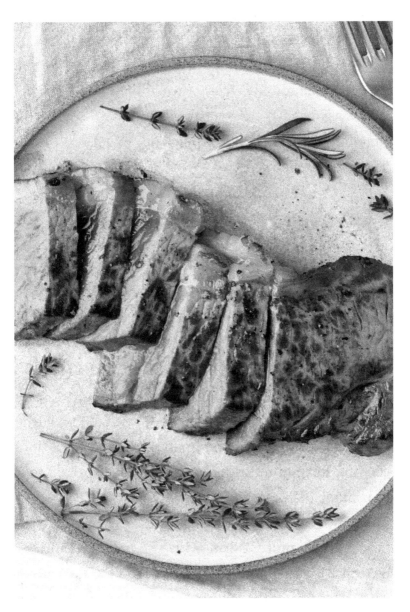

16 Easy Zucchini Beef Lasagna

Ready in about: 1 hour | Serves: 4

INGREDIENTS:

1 lb ground beef

2 large zucchinis, sliced lengthwise

3 cloves garlic

1 medium white onion, chopped

3 tomatoes, chopped

Salt and black pepper to taste

2 tsp sweet paprika

1 tsp dried thyme

1 tsp dried basil

1 cup mozzarella cheese, shredded

1 tbsp olive oil

DIRECTIONS:

Preheat the oven to 370°F. Heat the olive oil in a skillet over medium heat. Cook the beef for 4 minutes while breaking any lumps as you stir. Top with onion, garlic, tomatoes, salt, paprika, and pepper. Stir and continue cooking for 5 minutes. Lay ⅓ of the zucchini slices in the baking dish.

Top with ⅓ of the beef mixture and repeat the layering process two more times with the same quantities. Season with basil and thyme. Sprinkle the mozzarella cheese on top and tuck the baking dish in the oven.

Bake for 35 minutes. Remove the lasagna and let it rest for 10 minutes before serving.

NUTRITION: Cal 344, Fat 17.8g, Net Carbs 2.9g, Protein 40.4g

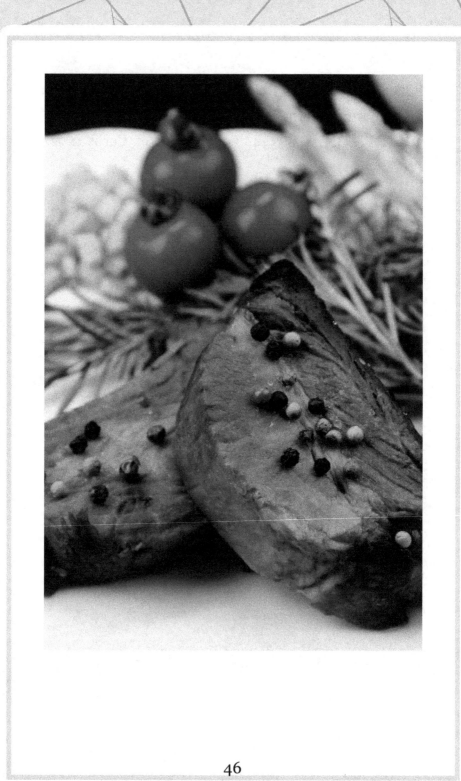

17 Rib Roast with Roasted Shallots & Garlic

Ready in about: 40 minutes | Serves: 6

INGREDIENTS:

5 lb beef rib roast, on the bone

3 heads garlic, cut in half

3 tbsp olive oil

6 shallots, peeled and halved

2 lemons, zested and juiced

3 tbsp mustard seeds

3 tbsp swerve

Salt and black pepper to taste

3 tbsp thyme leaves

DIRECTIONS:

Preheat oven to 400°F. Place garlic heads and shallots in a roasting dish, toss with olive oil, and bake for 15 minutes. Pour lemon juice on them. Score shallow crisscrosses patterns on the meat and set aside.

Mix swerve, mustard seeds, thyme, salt, pepper, and lemon zest to make a rub and apply it all over the beef. Place the beef on the shallots and garlic and cook in the oven for 20 minutes. Once ready, remove the dish, and let sit covered for 15 minutes before slicing. Serve.

NUTRITION: Cal 556, Fat 38.6g, Net Carbs 2.5g, Protein 58.4g

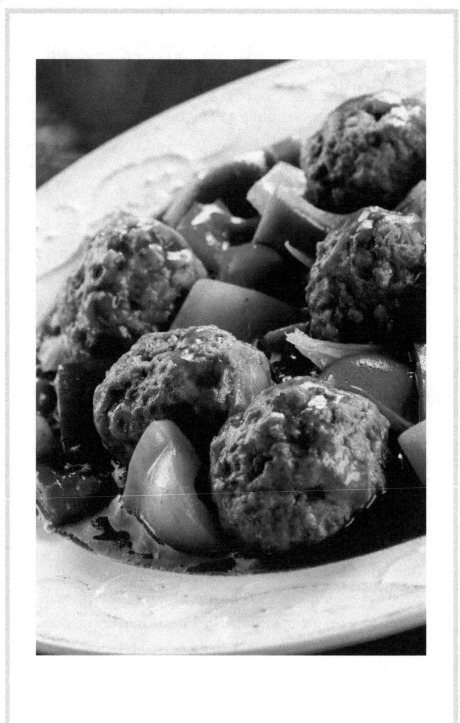

18 Habanero & Beef Balls

Ready in about: 45 minutes | Serves: 6

INGREDIENTS:

3 garlic cloves, minced

2 lb ground beef

1 onion, chopped

2 habanero peppers, chopped

1 tsp dried thyme

2 tsp fresh cilantro, chopped

½ tsp allspice

1 tsp cumin

½ tsp ground cloves

Salt and black pepper to taste

2 tbsp butter

3 tbsp butter, melted

6 oz cream cheese

1 tsp turmeric

¼ tsp stevia

½ tsp baking powder

1½ cups flax meal

½ cup coconut flour

DIRECTIONS:

In a blender, mix the onion with garlic, habaneros, and ½ cup water. Set a pan over medium heat, add 2 tbsp butter, and cook the beef for 3 minutes. Stir in the onion mixture, and cook for 2 minutes. Stir in cilantro, cloves, salt, cumin, turmeric, thyme, allspice, and pepper and cook for 3 minutes.

In a bowl, combine the coconut flour, stevia, flax meal, and baking powder and stir well. In a separate bowl, whisk the melted butter with the cream cheese. Mix the 2 mixtures to obtain a dough.

Form 12 balls from the mixture and roll them into circles. Split the beef mix on one-half of the dough circles, cover with the other half, seal edges, and lay on a lined sheet. Bake for 25 minutes in the oven at 350°F.

NUTRITION: Cal 455, Fat 31g, Net Carbs 8.3g, Protein 27g

19 Mustard-Lemon Beef

Ready in about: 25 minutes | Serves: 4

INGREDIENTS:

2 tbsp olive oil

1 tbsp fresh rosemary, chopped

2 garlic cloves, minced

1 ½ lb beef rump steak, thinly sliced

Salt and black pepper to taste

1 shallot, chopped

½ cup heavy cream

½ cup beef stock

1 tbsp mustard

2 tsp Worcestershire sauce

2 tsp lemon juice

1 tsp erythritol

2 tbsp butter

1 tbsp fresh rosemary, chopped

1 tbsp fresh thyme, chopped

DIRECTIONS:

In a bowl, combine 1 tbsp of oil with black pepper, garlic, rosemary, and salt. Toss in the beef to coat and set aside for some minutes. Heat a pan with the rest of the oil over medium heat, place in the beef steak, cook for 6 minutes, flipping halfway through. Set aside and keep warm.

Melt the butter in the pan. Add in the shallot and cook for 3 minutes. Stir in the stock, Worcestershire sauce, erythritol, thyme, cream, mustard, and rosemary and cook for 8 minutes. Mix in the lemon juice, pepper, and salt. Arrange the beef slices on serving plates, sprinkle over the sauce, and enjoy!

NUTRITION: Cal 435, Fat 30g, Net Carbs 5g, Protein 32g

20 Ribeye Steak with Shitake Mushrooms

Ready in about: 25 minutes | Serves: 4

INGREDIENTS:

1 lb ribeye steaks

1 tbsp butter

2 tbsp olive oil

1 cup shitake mushrooms, sliced

Salt and black pepper to taste

2 tbsp fresh parsley, chopped

DIRECTIONS:

Heat the olive oil in a pan over medium heat. Rub the steaks with salt and black pepper and cook about 4 minutes per side; reserve. Melt the butter in the pan and cook the shitakes for 4 minutes. Scatter the parsley over and pour the mixture over the steaks to serve.

NUTRITION: Cal 478, Fat: 31g, Net Carbs: 3g, Protein: 33g

Chapter 5. Lamb

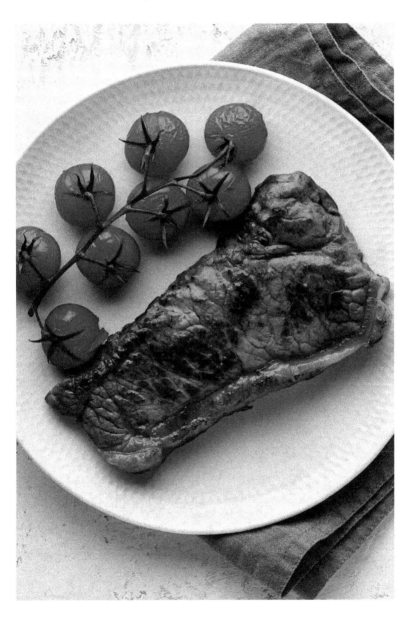

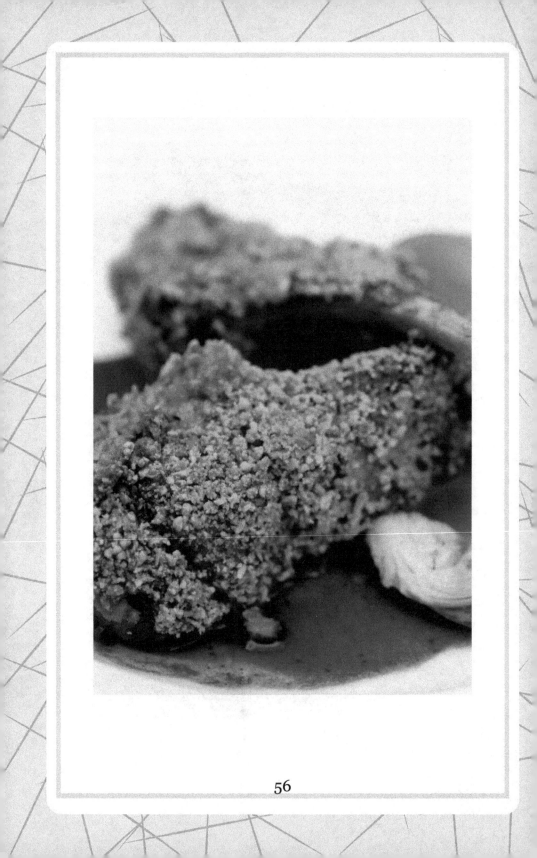

21 Grilled Lamb With Cream Mint Sauce

INGREDIENTS:

1 lamb (already marinated)

2 Tbsp chopped fresh dill

¼ cup minced fresh mint

2 Tbsp finely chopped red peppers

1 Tbsp lemon juice

1/8 cup coconut cream

DIRECTIONS:

Mix dill, mint, red pepper, lemon juice, and coconut cream. Chill until ready to serve

Turn on the grill; you want the lamb to be hot and brown quickly to keep the juice inside.

Chop on a hot grill and close the lid, cook approximately. 4 min

Using slippers (to keep the juice in, turn the top and cover for 4 min) Close for medium red, 6 for medium.

Pour over a generous portion of sauce and sprinkle.

NUTRITION: Cal 259 Fat: 12.6g, Net Carbs: 4.4g, Protein: 31g

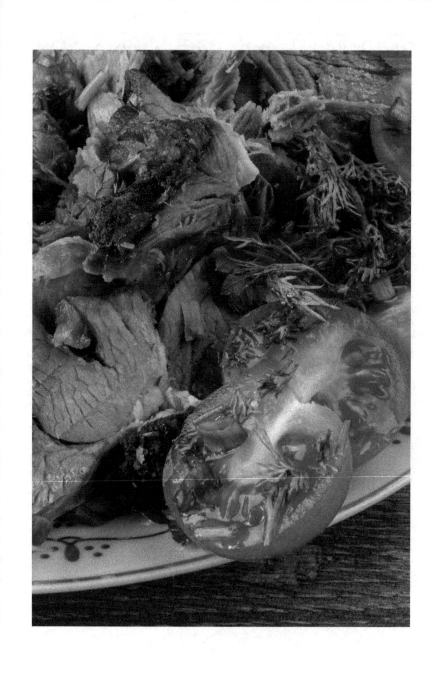

22 Lamb Roast with Tomatoes

Prep time: 10 minutes | Cook time: 7 to 8 hours | Serves 6

INGREDIENTS:

1 tablespoon extra-virgin olive oil

2 pounds (907 g) lamb shoulder roast

Salt, for seasoning

Freshly ground black pepper, for seasoning

1 (14.5-ounce / 411-g) can diced tomatoes

1 tablespoon cumin

2 teaspoons minced garlic

1 teaspoon paprika

1 teaspoon chili powder

1 cup sour cream

2 teaspoons chopped fresh parsley, for garnish

DIRECTIONS:

Lightly grease the insert of the slow cooker with the olive oil.

Lightly season the lamb with salt and pepper.

Place the lamb in the insert and add the tomatoes, cumin, garlic, paprika, and chili powder.

Cover and cook on low for 7 to 8 hours.

Stir in the sour cream.

Serve topped with the parsley.

NUTRITION: calories: 524 | fat: 43.1g | protein: 27.9g | carbs: 5.9g | net carbs: 4.9g | fiber: 1.0g

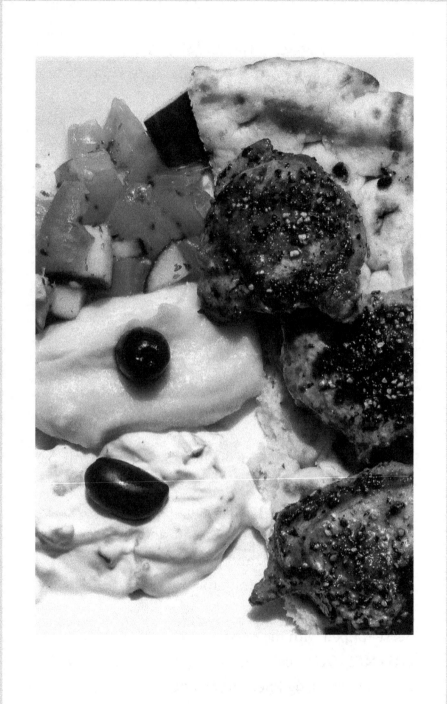

23 Greek Lamb Chops with Tzatziki Sauce

Prep time:10 min; Servings: 6

INGREDIENTS:

8 lamb chops

¼ cup lemon juice

2 Tbsp olive oil

1 shredded garlic clove

1½ tsp kosher salt

½ tsp pepper

Tzatziki sauce

2 cups natural Greek yogurt

2 cups cucumber in grated golden cubes

½ cup chopped fresh dill

¼ cup lemon juice

2 cloves garlic grated

½ tsp salt

¼ tsp pepper

DIRECTIONS:

Place the lamb chops on a large plate and dry with paper towels.

Mix lemon juice, olive oil, garlic, salt, and pepper in a large plastic bag with airtight seal or glass dish. Add chops to the wallet and seal. Move the bag to make sure the lamb chops are evenly coated with marinade — Marinate meat for 30 min or overnight.

Heat the grill over medium heat. Grill for 4 to 5 minutes per side or until meat thermometer reads 155 F. Remove from heat and leave for 10 min before serving. While the lamb is resting, prepare the Tzatziki sauce by combining all the ingredients in a medium-sized bowl. Check the herbs and adjust them accordingly. Serve the lamb chops with tzatziki sauce on the side.

NUTRITION: Cal 336 Carbs 8.5 g Protein 39.2 g Fat 15.9 g Saturated Fat 11.8 g

24 Lamb and Leek Burgers with Lemon Cream

INGREDIENTS:

For burgers:

45 g minced lamb

½ cup chopped leeks

1 Tbsp coconut oil, divided

½ Tbsp garlic powder.

½ tsp fine sea salt.

For the cream:

½ cup coconut cream

1 Tbsp lemon zest (1-2 lemons)

DIRECTIONS:

Put the chopped leeks and half of the coconut oil in a saucepan and cook over medium heat until the leeks soften about 3 to 5 min, put the leeks and let them cool down.

Place the ground lamb, garlic powder, and salt in a second large pot. Once the leeks are no longer hot, place the leeks to the bowl and gently mix until smooth mixture. Divide into 4 patties.

Put the rest of the coconut oil in a saucepan. Add the patties over medium heat and cook the golden brown on each side, about 5 min on each side. Make sure the lamb is cooked through.

NUTRITION: Cal 150 Fat: 6g, Net Carbs: 4.8g, Protein: 21g

25 Van Lamb with Roasted Tomatoes

Prep time:25 min; Servings: 5

INGREDIENTS:

For the lamb

2 ribs of lamb (trimmed in French, 4 lamb chops per person)

1 cup macadamia nuts

1 large garlic clove, peeled

½ cup chopped parsley

4 Tbsp olive oil

2/3 tsp sea salt

a little salt and black pepper

Golden Ghee or coconut oil

large roasting pan

For tomatoes

2 cherry tomatoes

2 Tbsp olive oil

2 Tbsp balsamic vinegar

½ tsp sea salt

DIRECTIONS:

Preheat oven to 170 C / 335 F to make roasted tomatoes. Place the cherry tomatoes on a roasting dish and sprinkle with olive oil.

Bake in the oven on the middle rack for 30 min Remove from the oven, sprinkle with balsamic vinegar, and put back in the oven for 10-15 min Remove the dish and sprinkle the tomatoes with sea salt. Set aside.

To make lamb, wash and dry the lamb chops.

Place the macadamia nuts, chopped parsley, and a clove of garlic in a food processor.

Add 4 Tbsp olive oil and a generous pinch of salt.

Heat Ghee or coconut oil in a saucepan. Place lamb chops for 1 minute. Turn the boards over and cook another minute on each side of the layer of macadamia pasta 0.5 cm thick, press with your fingers. Place in the refrigerator for 10 min

The lamb grilled on a lightly greased baking belt, cut and bake for 12 min at 200 ° C / 390 ° F. Bake at 170 ° C / 335 ° F and bake again with a duration of 8 to 10 min

Preheat the oven to 200 ° C / 390 ° F.

Let the oven rest for 5 min before serving. The crust is a little fragile, but also cautious when transferring the lamb in a serving dish. I cut the grates in half to help them effectively on 4 scales. Place the roasted tomatoes around the lamb.

NUTRITION: Cal 359 Fat: 16.4g, Net Carbs: 30.5g, Protein: 27.2g

Chapter 6. Pork Recipes

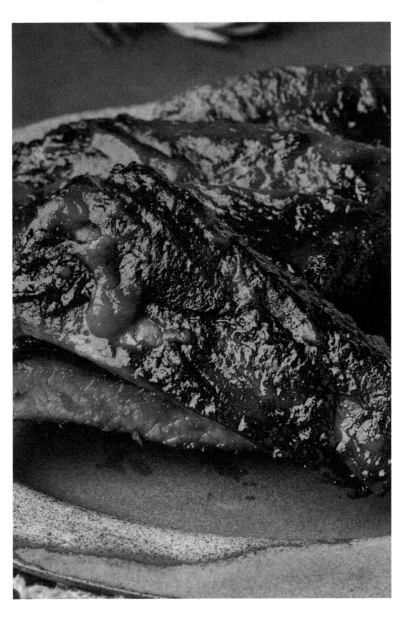

26 Pork Wraps

Ready in about: 40 minutes | Serves: 6

NUTRITION: Cal 435, Fat 37g, Net Carbs 2g, Protein 34g

Ingredients

6 bacon slices

2 tbsp fresh parsley, chopped

1 lb pork tenderloin, sliced

⅓ cup ricotta cheese

3 tbsp coconut oil

¼ cup onions, chopped

3 garlic cloves, minced

2 tbsp Parmesan cheese, grated

15 oz canned diced tomatoes

⅓ cup vegetable stock

Salt and black pepper to taste

½ tsp Italian seasoning

DIRECTIONS:

Use a meat pounder to flatten the pork pieces. Set the bacon slices on top of each piece and divide the parsley, ricotta cheese, and Parmesan cheese between them. Roll each pork piece and secure it with a toothpick. Set a pan over medium heat and warm oil. Cook the pork rolls until browned. Remove.

Add onions and garlic in the pan and cook for 5 minutes. Place in the stock and cook for 3 minutes. Get rid of the toothpicks from the rolls and return to the pan. Stir in pepper, salt, tomatoes, and Italian seasoning. Bring to a boil, reduce the heat, and cook for 20 minutes covered. Split among bowls to serve.

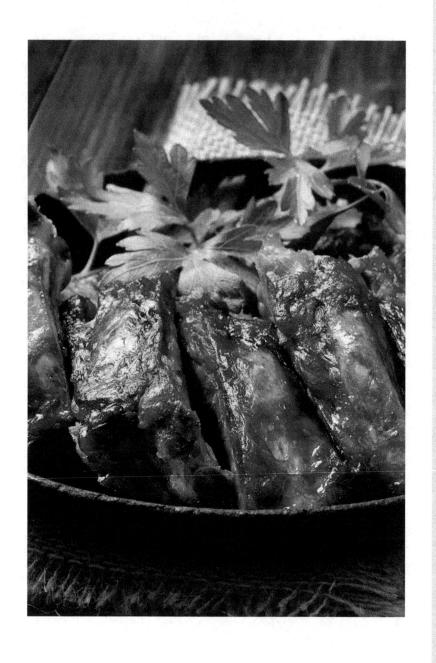

27 Spicy Pork Ribs

Ready in about: 8 hours 45 minutes | Serves: 6

NUTRITION: Cal 580, Fat 36.6g, Net Carbs 0g, Protein 44.5g

Ingredients

3 racks pork ribs, silver lining removed

2 cups sugar-free BBQ sauce

2 tbsp erythritol

2 tsp chili powder

2 tsp cumin powder

2 tsp smoked paprika

2 tsp garlic powder

Salt and black pepper to taste

1 tsp mustard powder

DIRECTIONS:

Preheat a smoker to 400°F, using mesquite wood to create flavor in the smoker. In a bowl, mix the erythritol, chili powder, cumin powder, black pepper, smoked paprika, garlic powder, salt, and mustard powder. Rub the ribs and let marinate for 30 minutes. Place on the grill grate and cook at reduced heat of 225°F for 4 hours. Flip the ribs after and continue cooking for 4 hours. Brush the ribs with bbq sauce on both sides and sear them in increased heat for 3 minutes per side. Remove and let sit for 4 minutes before slicing. Serve with red cabbage coleslaw.

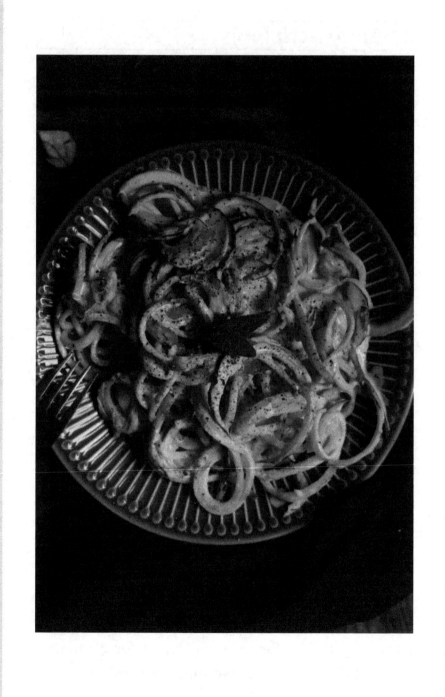

28 Zoodle & Bacon Halloumi Gratin with Spinach

Ready in about: 35 minutes | Serves: 4

NUTRITION: Cal 350, Fat 27g, Net Carbs 5.3g, Protein 16g

Ingredients

2 large zucchinis, spiralized

4 slices bacon, chopped

2 cups baby spinach

4 oz halloumi cheese, cut into cubes

2 cloves garlic, minced

1 cup heavy cream

½ cup sugar-free tomato sauce

1 cup mozzarella cheese, grated

½ tsp dried Italian herbs

DIRECTIONS:

Preheat oven to 350°F. Place a pan over medium heat and fry the bacon for 4 minutes. Add in the garlic and cook for 1 minute. In a bowl, mix heavy cream, tomato sauce, and 1/6 cup water and add it to the pan.

Stir in zucchini, spinach, halloumi, Italian herbs, salt, and pepper. Sprinkle the mozzarella cheese on top and transfer the pan to the oven. Bake for 20 minutes or until the cheese is golden. Serve warm.

29 Pancetta & Kale Pork Sausages

Ready in about: 30 minutes | Serves: 4

NUTRITION: Cal 386, Fat 29g, Net Carbs 5.4g, Protein2 1g

Ingredients

2 cups kale

4 cups chicken vegetable broth

2 tbsp olive oil

1 cup heavy cream

3 pancetta slices, chopped

½ lb radishes, chopped

2 garlic cloves, minced

Salt and black pepper to taste

½ tsp red pepper flakes

1 onion, chopped

1 ½ lb hot pork sausage, chopped

DIRECTIONS:

Warm the olive oil in a pot over medium heat. Stir in garlic, onion, pancetta, and sausage and cook for 5 minutes. Pour in the vegetable broth, radishes, and kale and simmer for 10 minutes. Sprinkle with salt, red pepper flakes, and black pepper. Add in the heavy cream, stir, and cook for about 5 minutes. Serve.

30 Pork Lettuce Cups

Ready in about: 20 minutes | Serves: 6

NUTRITION: Cal 311, Fat 24.3g, Net Carbs 1g, Protein 19g

Ingredients

2 lb ground pork

1 tbsp ginger-garlic paste

Pink salt and black pepper to taste

3 tbsp butter

Leaves from 1 head Iceberg lettuce

2 green onions, chopped

1 red bell pepper, chopped

½ cucumber, finely chopped

½ tsp cayenne pepper

DIRECTIONS:

Melt butter in a pan over medium heat. Rub the pork with ginger-garlic paste, salt, pepper, and cayenne pepper and add it to the pan. Cook for 10 minutes until the pork is no longer pink. Remove and let it cool.

Pat the lettuce leaves dry with paper towels. Spoon two to three tablespoons of the pork mixture in each leaf. Top with green onions, bell pepper, and cucumber. Serve with soy drizzling sauce.

Chapter 7. Fish and Seafood

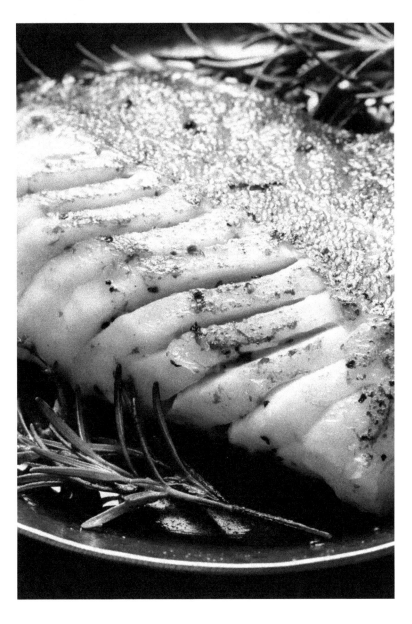

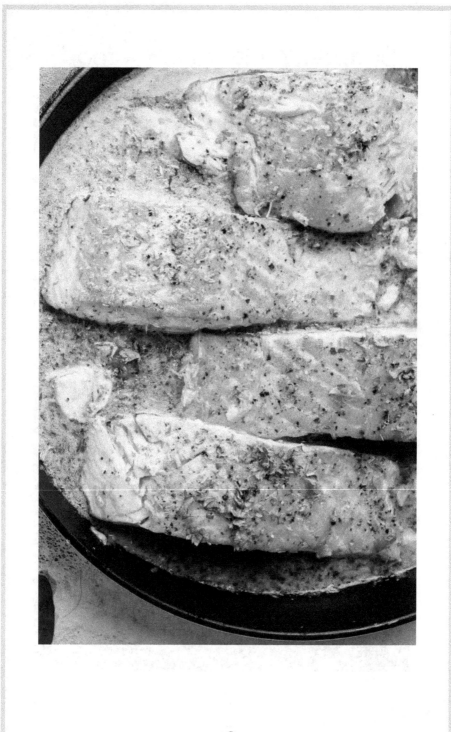

31 Sour Cream Salmon with Parmesan

Ready in about: 25 minutes | Serves: 4

INGREDIENTS:

1 cup sour cream

1 tbsp fresh dill, chopped

½ lemon, zested and juiced

Pink Salt and black pepper to taste

4 salmon steaks

½ cup Parmesan cheese, grated

DIRECTIONS:

Preheat oven to 400°F. In a bowl, mix the sour cream, dill, lemon zest, juice, salt, and pepper. Season the fish with salt and black pepper, drizzle lemon juice on both sides of the fish, and arrange them on a lined baking sheet. Spread the sour cream mixture on each fish and sprinkle with Parmesan cheese.

Bake the fish for 15 minutes and after broil the top for 2 minutes with a close watch for a nice brown color. Plate the fish and serve with buttery green beans.

NUTRITION: Cal 288, Fat 23.4g, Net Carbs 1.2g, Protein 16.2g

32 Tilapia with Olives & Tomato Sauce

Ready in about: 30 minutes | Serves: 4

INGREDIENTS:

4 tilapia fillets

2 garlic cloves, minced

½ tsp dried oregano

14 oz canned tomatoes, diced

2 tbsp olive oil

½ red onion, chopped

2 tbsp fresh parsley, chopped

¼ cup Kalamata olives

DIRECTIONS:

Heat olive oil in a skillet over medium heat and cook the onion for 3 minutes. Add garlic and oregano and cook for 30 seconds. Stir in tomatoes and bring the mixture to a boil. Reduce the heat and simmer for 5 minutes. Add olives and tilapia and cook for about 8 minutes. Serve the tilapia with tomato sauce.

NUTRITION: Cal 282, Fat: 15g, Net Carbs: 6g, Protein: 23g

33 Seared Scallops with Chorizo and Asiago Cheese

Ready in about: 15 minutes | Serves: 4

INGREDIENTS:

2 tbsp ghee

16 fresh scallops

8 oz chorizo, chopped

1 red bell pepper, seeds removed, sliced

1 cup red onions, finely chopped

1 cup asiago cheese, grated

Salt and black pepper to taste

DIRECTIONS:

Melt half of the ghee in a skillet over medium heat, and cook the onion and bell pepper for 5 minutes until tender. Add the chorizo and stir-fry for another 3 minutes. Remove and set aside.

Pat dry the scallops with paper towels and season with salt and pepper. Add the remaining ghee to the skillet and sear the scallops for 2 minutes on each side to have a golden brown color. Add the chorizo mixture back and warm through. Transfer to serving platter and top with asiago cheese.

NUTRITION: Cal 491, Fat 32g, Net Carbs 5g, Protein 36g

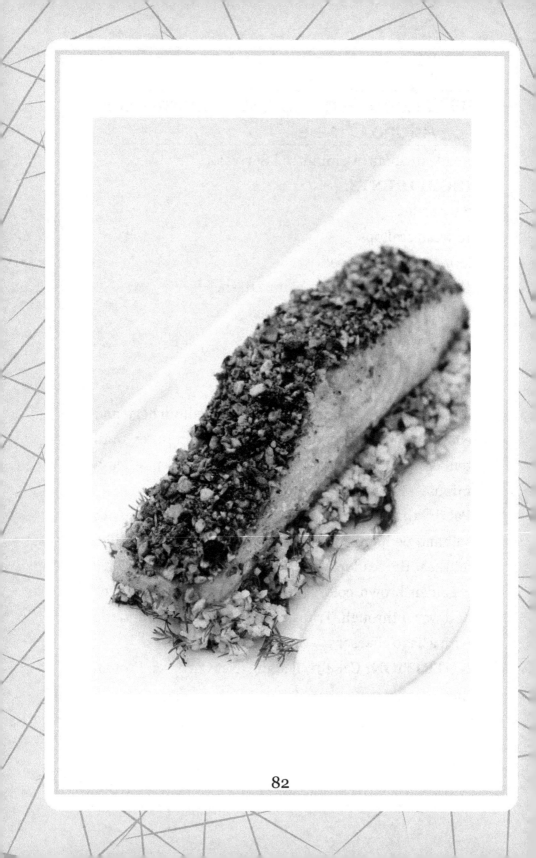

34 Pistachio-Crusted Salmon

Ready in about: 25 minutes | Serves: 4

INGREDIENTS:

4 salmon fillets

Salt and black pepper to taste

¼ cup mayonnaise

½ cup chopped pistachios

1 shallot, chopped

2 tsp lemon zest

2 tbsp olive oil

1 cup heavy cream

DIRECTIONS:

Preheat oven to 370°F. Brush the salmon with mayonnaise and season with salt and pepper. Coat with pistachios, place in a lined baking dish, and bake for 15 minutes. Heat olive oil in a saucepan and sauté the shallot for 3 minutes. Stir in the rest of the ingredients. Cook until thickened, 10 minutes. Serve.

NUTRITION: Cal 563, Fat: 47g, Net Carbs: 6g, Protein: 34g

35 Cod in Garlic Butter Sauce

Ready in about: 20 minutes | Serves: 6

INGREDIENTS:

2 tsp olive oil

6 Alaska cod fillets

Salt and black pepper to taste

4 tbsp butter

3 cloves garlic, minced

⅓ cup lemon juice

3 tbsp white wine

2 tbsp chopped chives

DIRECTIONS:

Heat the oil in a skillet over medium heat. Season the cod with salt and black pepper. Fry the fillets in the oil for 4 minutes on one side, flip, and cook for 1 minute. Take out, plate, and set aside.

In the same skillet over, melt the butter and sauté the garlic for 3 minutes. Add the lemon juice, white wine, and chives. Season with salt and black pepper and cook for 3 minutes until the wine **NUTRITION:** Cal 264, Fat 17.3g, Net Carbs 2.3g, Protein 20g

slightly reduces. Put the fish in a platter, spoon the sauce over, and serve with buttered green beans.

Chapter 8. Salad Recipes

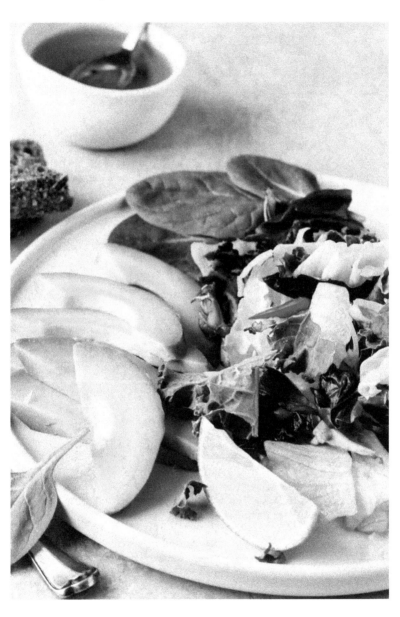

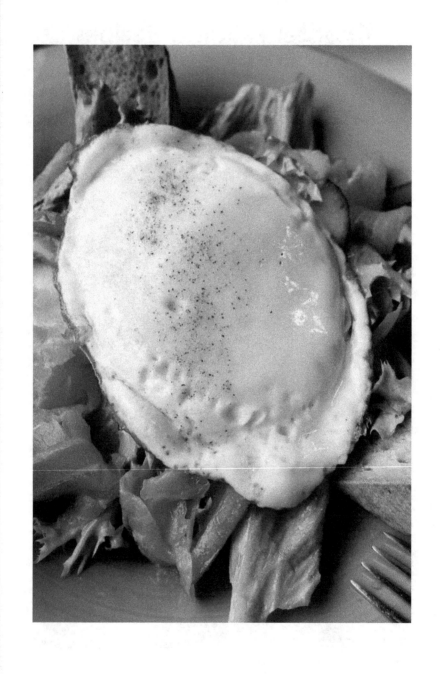

36 Caesar Salad with Smoked Salmon & Poached Eggs

Ready in about: 15 minutes | Serves: 4

INGREDIENTS:

3 cups water

8 eggs

2 cups torn romaine lettuce

½ cup smoked salmon, chopped

6 slices bacon

2 tbsp low carb Caesar dressing

DIRECTIONS:

Boil the water in a pot over medium heat for 5 minutes and bring to simmer. Crack each egg into a small bowl and gently slide into the water. Poach for 2 to 3 minutes, remove with a perforated spoon, transfer to a paper towel to dry, and plate. Poach the remaining 7 eggs.

Put the bacon in a skillet and fry over medium heat until browned and crispy, about 6 minutes, turning once. Remove, allow cooling, and chop into small pieces. Toss the lettuce, smoked salmon, bacon, and Caesar dressing in a salad bowl. Top with two eggs each and serve immediately or chilled.

NUTRITION: Cal 260, Fat 21g, Net Carbs 5g, Protein 8g

37 Chicken Salad with Grapefruit & Cashews

Ready in about: 30 minutes + marinating time|

Serves: 4

INGREDIENTS:

1 grapefruit, peeled and segmented

1 chicken breast

4 green onions, sliced

10 oz baby spinach

2 tbsp cashews

1 red chili pepper, thinly sliced

1 lemon, juiced

3 tbsp olive oil

Salt and black pepper to taste

DIRECTIONS:

Toast the cashews in a dry pan over high heat for 2 minutes, shaking often. Set aside to cool, then chop. Preheat the grill to medium heat. Season the chicken with salt and pepper and brush with some olive oil. Grill for 4 minutes per side. Remove to a plate and let it sit for a few minutes before slicing.

Place the baby spinach and green onions on a serving platter. Season with salt, remaining olive oil, and lemon juice. Toss to coat. Top with chicken, chili pepper, and chicken. Sprinkle with cashews and serve.

NUTRITION: Cal 178, Fat: 13.5g, Net Carbs: 3.2g, Protein: 9.1g

38 Mediterranean Tomato and Zucchini Salad

Prep time: 15 minutes | Cook time: 10 minutes | Serves 4

INGREDIENTS:

½ pound (227 g) Roma tomatoes, sliced

½ pound (227 g) zucchini, sliced

1 Lebanese cucumber, sliced

1 cup arugula

½ teaspoon oregano

½ teaspoon basil

½ teaspoon rosemary

½ teaspoon ground black pepper

Sea salt, to season

4 tablespoons extra-virgin olive oil

2 tablespoons fresh lemon juice

½ cup Kalamata olives, pitted and sliced

4 ounces (113 g) Feta cheese, cubed

DIRECTIONS:

Arrange the Roma tomatoes and zucchini slices on a roasting pan; spritz cooking oil over your vegetables.

Bake in the preheated oven at 350°F (180°C) for 6 to 7 minutes. Let them cool slightly, then, transfer to a salad bowl.

Add in the cucumber, arugula, herbs, and spices. Drizzle olive oil and lemon juice over your veggies; toss to combine well.

Top with Kalamata olives and Feta cheese. Serve at room temperature and enjoy!

NUTRITION:

calories: 242 | fat: 22.1g | protein: 6.4g | carbs: 6.9g | net carbs: 5.1g | fiber: 1.8g

39 Grilled Steak Salad with Pickled Peppers

Ready in about: 15 minutes | Serves: 4

INGREDIENTS:

½ lb skirt steak, sliced

Salt and black pepper to taste

3 tsp olive oil

1 head Romaine lettuce, torn

3 chopped pickled peppers

2 tbsp red wine vinegar

½ cup queso fresco, crumbled

1 tbsp green olives, pitted, sliced

DIRECTIONS:

Brush the steak slices with some olive oil and season with salt and black pepper on both sides. Heat a grill pan over high heat and cook the steaks on each side for about 5-6 minutes. Remove to a bow.

Mix the lettuce, pickled peppers, remaining olive oil, and vinegar in a salad bowl. Add the beef and sprinkle with queso fresco and green olives. Serve.

NUTRITION: Cal 315, Fat 26g, Net Carbs 2g, Protein 18g

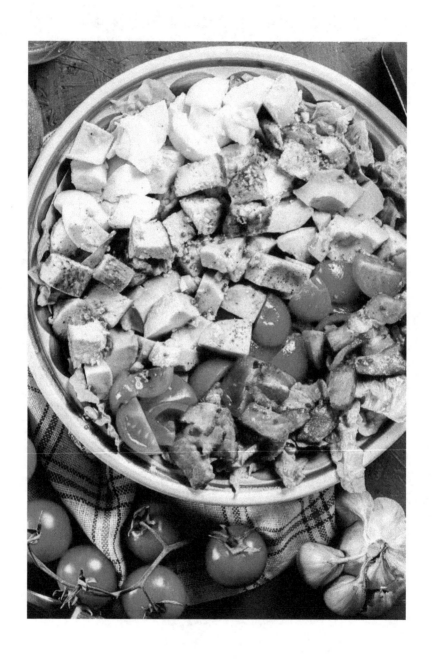

40 Cobb Salad with Blue Cheese Dressing

Ready in about: 30 minutes | Serves: 6

INGREDIENTS:

Dressing

½ cup buttermilk

1 cup mayonnaise

2 tbsp Worcestershire sauce

½ cup sour cream

1 cup blue cheese, crumbled

2 tbsp chives, chopped

Salad

6 eggs

2 chicken breasts

5 strips bacon

1 iceberg lettuce, cut into chunks

Salt and black pepper to taste

1 romaine lettuce, chopped

1 bibb lettuce, cored, leaves removed

2 avocado, pitted and diced

2 large tomatoes, chopped

½ cup blue cheese, crumbled

2 scallions, chopped

DIRECTIONS:

In a bowl, whisk the buttermilk, mayonnaise, Worcestershire sauce, and sour cream. Stir in the blue cheese and chives. Place in the refrigerator to chill until ready to use. Bring the eggs to boil in salted water over medium heat for 10 minutes. Transfer to an ice bath to cool. Peel and chop. Set aside.

Preheat a grill pan over high heat. Season the chicken with salt and pepper. Grill for 3 minutes on each side. Remove to a plate to cool for 3 minutes and cut into bite-size chunks. Fry the bacon in the same pan until crispy, about 6 minutes. Remove, let cool for 2 minutes, and chop.

Arrange the lettuce leaves in a salad bowl, and in single piles, add the avocado, tomatoes, eggs, bacon, and chicken. Sprinkle the blue cheese over the salad as well as the scallions and black pepper. Drizzle the blue cheese dressing on the salad and serve with low carb bread.

NUTRITION: Cal 122, Fat 14g, Net Carbs 2g, Protein 23g

Chapter 9. Soup Recipes

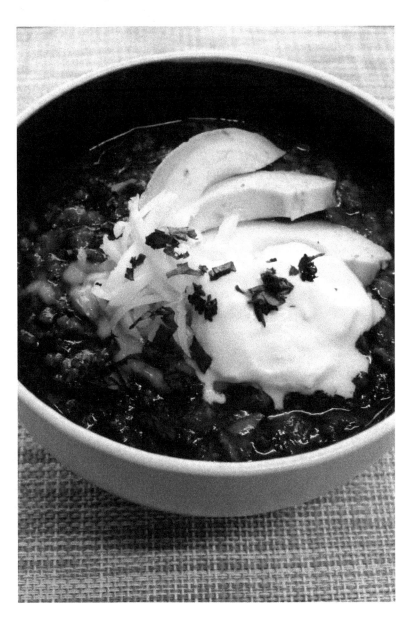

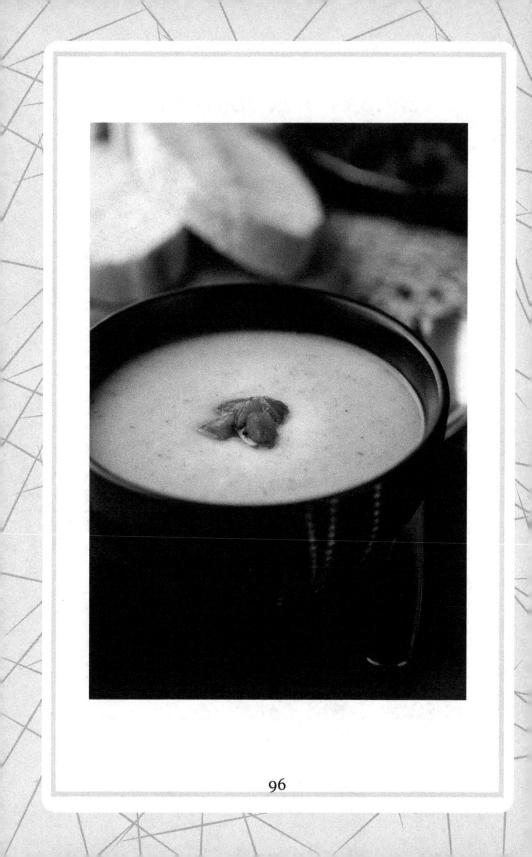

41 Cauliflower Soup with Kielbasa

Total Time: approx. 35 minutes|4 servings

INGREDIENTS:

1 cauliflower head, chopped

1 rutabaga, chopped

3 tbsp ghee

1 kielbasa sausage, sliced

2 cups chicken broth

1 small onion, chopped

2 cups water

Salt and black pepper, to taste

DIRECTIONS:

Melt the ghee in a pot over medium heat and cook kielbasa sausage for 5 minutes; reserve. Add onion to the pot and sauté for 3 minutes. Add in cauliflower and rutabaga and cook for another 5 minutes. Pour in broth, water, salt, and pepper. Bring to a boil and simmer for 15 minutes. Puree the soup until smooth. Serve topped with kielbasa.

NUTRITION: Cal 251; Net Carbs: 5g; Fat: 19g, Protein: 10g

42 Colby Cauliflower Soup with Pancetta Chips

Total Time: approx. 30 minutes|4 servings

INGREDIENTS:

1 head cauliflower, cut into florets

2 tbsp ghee

1 onion, chopped

2 cups water

3 cups almond milk

1 cup Colby cheese, shredded

3 pancetta strips

Salt and black pepper to taste

DIRECTIONS:

Melt ghee in a saucepan over medium heat and sauté onion for 3 minutes. Include cauli florets and cook for 3 minutes. Add in water and season with salt and pepper. Bring to a boil and simmer for 10 minutes. Puree the soup and stir in almond milk and Colby cheese until the cheese melts. In a skillet over medium heat, fry pancetta until crispy. Top the soup with pancetta and ladle into bowls to serve.

NUTRITION: Cal 402; Net Carbs 6g; Fat 37g; Protein 8g

43 Asparagus & Shrimp Curry Soup

Total Time: approx. 20 minutes|4 servings

INGREDIENTS:

2 tbsp ghee

1 lb jumbo shrimp, deveined

2 tsp ginger-garlic puree

2 tbsp red curry paste

1 cup coconut milk

1 bunch asparagus

DIRECTIONS:

Melt ghee in a saucepan over medium heat and add in the shrimp. Sauté for 3 minutes; remove to a plate. Add ginger-garlic puree and red curry paste to the saucepan and cook for 2 minutes. Stir in coconut milk and 3 cups water. Add the shrimp and asparagus. Cook for 4 minutes. Reduce the heat and simmer for 3 more minutes. Serve.

NUTRITION: Cal 375; Net Carbs 2g; Fat 35.4g, Protein 9g

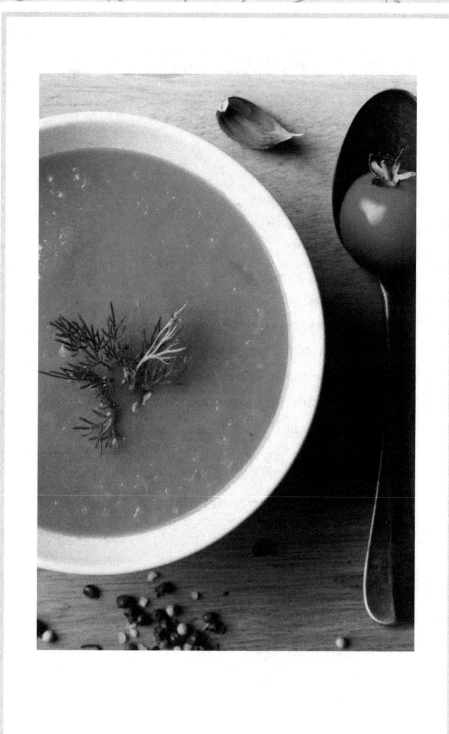

44 Thyme Tomato Soup

Total Time: approx. 20 minutes|6 servings

INGREDIENTS:

2 tbsp butter

2 large red onions, diced

½ cup raw cashew nuts, diced

2 (28-oz) cans tomatoes

1 tsp thyme

1 ½ cups water

Salt and black pepper to taste

1 cup half-and-half

DIRECTIONS:

Melt butter in a pot over medium heat and sauté the onion for 4 minutes. Stir in tomatoes, thyme, water, cashews, salt, and pepper. Bring to a boil and simmer for 10 minutes. Puree the ingredients with an immersion blender. Stir in half-and-half. Spoon into soup bowls and serve warm.

NUTRITION: Cal 310; Net Carbs 3g; Fat 27g, Protein 11g

45 Coconut Turkey Chili

Total Time: approx. 25 minutes|4 servings

INGREDIENTS:

1 lb turkey breasts, cubed

1 cup broccoli, chopped

2 shallots, sliced

1 (14-oz) can tomatoes

2 tbsp coconut oil

2 tbsp coconut cream

2 garlic cloves, minced

1 tbsp ground coriander

2 tbsp fresh ginger, grated

1 tbsp turmeric

1 tbsp cumin

2 tbsp chili powder

DIRECTIONS:

Melt coconut oil in a pan over medium heat and stir-fry turkey, shallots, garlic, and ginger for 5 minutes. Stir in tomatoes, broccoli, turmeric, coriander, cumin, and chili. Pour in coconut cream and cook for 15 minutes. Transfer to a food processor and blend well. Serve warm.

NUTRITION: Cal 318; Net Carbs 6.6g; Fat 18g; Protein 27g

Chapter 10. Dessert Recipes

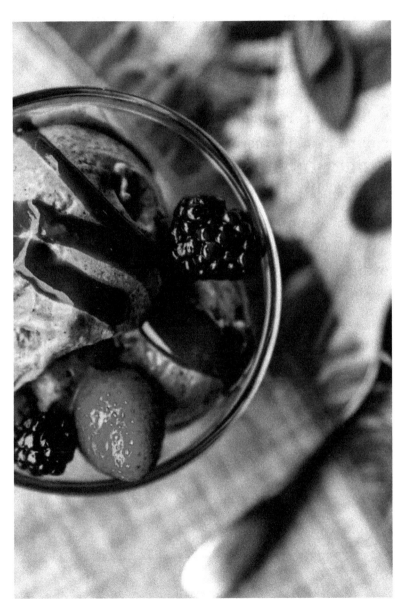

46 Ricotta Parfait with Strawberries

Total Time: approx. 10 minutes|4 servings

INGREDIENTS:

1 cup ricotta cheese

2 cups strawberries, chopped

2 tbsp sugar-free maple syrup

2 tbsp balsamic vinegar

DIRECTIONS:

Distribute half of the strawberries between 4 small glasses and top with ricotta cheese.

Drizzle with maple syrup, balsamic vinegar and finish with the remaining strawberries.

Serve.

NUTRITION: Cal 159; Net Carbs 3.1g; Fats 8g; Protein 6.9g

47 Cream Mousse

Prep time: 10 minutes | Cook time: 0 minutes | Serves 4

INGREDIENTS:

2 cups double cream

4 egg yolks

½ teaspoon instant coffee

1 teaspoon pure coconut extract

6 tablespoons Xylitol

DIRECTIONS:

Heat the cream in a pan over low heat; let it cool slightly.

Then, whisk the egg yolks with the instant coffee, coconut extract, and Xylitol until well combined.

Add the egg mixture to the lukewarm cream. Warm the mixture over low heat until it has reduced and thickened.

Refrigerate for 3 hours before serving. Enjoy!

NUTRITION: Cal: 290 | fat: 27.7g | protein: 6.0g | carbs: 5.0g | net carbs: 5.0g | fiber: 0g

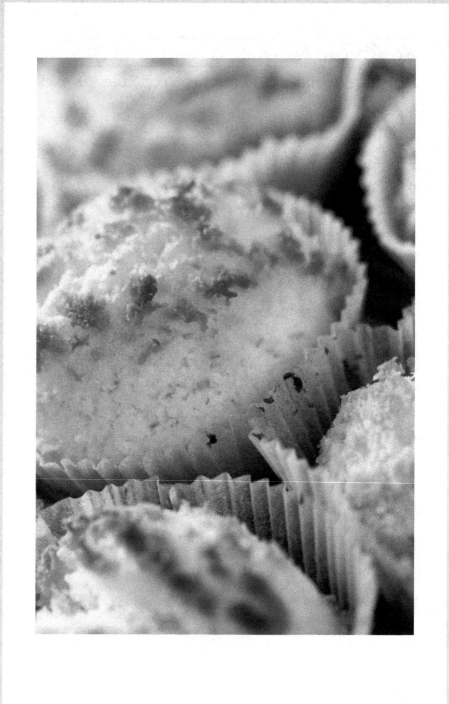

48 Super Coconut Cupcakes

Prep time: 15 minutes | Cook time: 15 minutes | Serves 9

INGREDIENTS:

6 eggs, beaten

½ cup coconut oil, melted

3 tablespoons granulated Swerve

2 tablespoons flaxseed meal

⅓ cup coconut flour

1 teaspoon baking powder

A pinch of salt

A pinch of freshly grated nutmeg

1 teaspoon lemon zest

1 teaspoon coconut extract

DIRECTIONS:

Start by preheating your oven to 360°F (182°C). Coat a muffin pan with cupcake liners.

Beat the eggs with the coconut oil and granulated Swerve until frothy. In another mixing bowl, thoroughly combine the remaining ingredients.

Stir this dry mixture into the wet mixture; mix again to combine. Spoon the batter into the prepared muffin pan.

Bake for 13 to 15 minutes, or until a tester comes out dry and clean. To serve, sprinkle with some extra granulated Swerve if desired. Bon appétit!

NUTRITION: Cal: 164 | fat: 16.8g | protein: 2.2g | carbs: 1.6g | net carbs: 0.7g | fiber: 0.9g

49 Penuche Bars

Prep time: 15 minutes | Cook time: 0 minutes | Serves 10

INGREDIENTS:

½ stick butter

2 tablespoons tahini (sesame paste)

½ cup almond butter

1 teaspoon Stevia

2 ounces (57 g) baker's chocolate, sugar-free

A pinch of salt

A pinch of grated nutmeg

½ teaspoon cinnamon powder

DIRECTIONS:

Microwave the butter for 30 to 35 seconds. Fold in the tahini, almond butter, Stevia, and chocolate.

Sprinkle with salt, nutmeg, and cinnamon; whisk to combine well. Scrape the mixture into a parchment-lined baking tray.

Transfer to the freezer for 40 minutes. Cut into bars and enjoy!

NUTRITION: Cal: 180 | fat: 18.4g | protein: 1.7g | carbs: 3.1g | net carbs: 2.0g | fiber: 1.1g

50 Creamy Avocado Custard

INGREDIENTS: 4 servings

3 soft avocados

2 tsp agar powder

½ cup heavy cream

½ lime, juiced

½ cup water

Salt and black pepper to taste

DIRECTIONS: and Total Time: approx. 10 min + chilling time

Place ¼ cup of the water in a bowl and sprinkle agar powder on top; set aside to dissolve.

Core, peel avocados, and add the flesh to a food processor.

Top with heavy cream, lime juice, salt, and pepper.

Process until smooth and pour in agar liquid.

Blend further until smooth.

Divide the mixture between 4 ramekins and chill overnight.

NUTRITION: Cal 302; Net Carbs 7.9g; Fat 27g; Protein 2.9g

CPSIA information can be obtained
at www.ICGtesting.com
Printed in the USA
LVHW011113090621
689683LV00010B/912

9 781803 214603